The Fabian Society is Britain's oldest political think tank. Since 1884 the society has played a central role in developing political ideas and public policy on the left.

Through a wide range of publications and events the society influences political and public thinking, but also provides a space for broad and open-minded debate, drawing on an unrivalled external network and its own expert research and analysis.

The society is alone among think tanks in being a democratically-constituted membership organisation, with over 7,000 members. During its history the membership has included many of the key thinkers on the British left and every Labour prime minister. Today it counts over 200 parliamentarians in its number. Member-led activity includes 70 local Fabian societies, the Scottish and Welsh Fabians, the Fabian Women's Network and the Young Fabians, which is itself the leading organisation on the left for young people to debate and influence political ideas.

The society was one of the original founders of the Labour party and is constitutionally affiliated to the party. It is however editorially, organisationally and financially independent and works with a wide range of partners of all political persuasions and none.

Fabian Society
61 Petty France
London SW1H 9EU
www.fabians.org.uk

Fabian Ideas 646

First published July 2018
ISBN 978-0-7163-0646-7

Editorial director: Kate Murray
Editorial assistant: Vanesha Singh

*This pamphlet, like all publications of the Fabian Society,
represents not the collective views of the society but only the
views of the authors. The responsibility of the society is limited
to approving its publications as worthy of consideration within
the Labour movement. This publication may not be reproduced
without express permission of the Fabian Society.*

Printed and bound by DG3, London, UK

To find out more about the Fabian Society, the Young
Fabians, the Fabian Women's Network and our local
societies, please visit our website at www.fabians.org.uk

A picture of health

The NHS at 70 and its future

Edited by Jonathan Ashworth MP

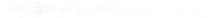

Project partners

SANOFI 🌀 *Empowering Life*

Supported by a grant from Sanofi. This pamphlet was created independently and Sanofi has no editorial control over its contents.

Sanofi, a global healthcare leader. Discovers, develops and distributes therapeutic solutions focused on patients' needs. Sanofi has core strengths in innovative drugs in diabetes, cardiovascular disease, rare diseases, multiple sclerosis, human vaccines and consumer healthcare. safoni.co.uk

UNISON – the public service union – serves over 1.3 million members and is the leading union for heath staff in the UK.

About the authors

Jonathan Ashworth is the Labour and Co-operative MP for Leicester South and the shadow health secretary.

Luciana Berger is the Labour and Co-operative MP for Liverpool Wavertree, president of the Labour Campaign for Mental Health, and a member of the health & social care select committee.

Tara Donnelly is chief executive at the Health Innovation Network, an organisation which has no political affiliations.

Sara Gorton is head of health at UNISON.

Chris Graham is chief executive of Picker, a charity that exists to promote and improve person-centred care. He oversaw the development of the NHS staff and patient survey programmes on behalf of NHS England and the Care Quality Commission respectively.

Kevin Gulliver is director of the Human City Institute, which is a Birmingham-based research charity and think tank.

Andrew Harrop is general secretary of the Fabian Society.

Lord Kerslake is former head of the civil service and current president of the Local Government Association. He stood down from his role as chairman of King's College hospital, London last year.

John Lister is information director at London Health Emergency and co-chair of Keep Our NHS Public. He was an associate senior lecturer in health policy and in journalism and health journalism at Coventry University.

Neena Modi is professor of neonatal medicine at Imperial College London and immediate past-president of the Royal College of Paediatrics and Child Health.

Dr Stephanie Snow is director of NHS at 70: The Story of Our Lives and Wellcome Trust University Award holder at the University of Manchester's centre for the history of science, technology & medicine.

Paul Williams is the Labour MP for Stockton South and a GP.

CONTENTS

INTRODUCTION

Jonathan Ashworth MP

WB Yeats wrote that 'in dreams begins responsibility'. When it comes to the National Health Service, Labour's proudest and most enduring achievement, that dream began with the Fabian Society. It was Beatrice Webb, in her minority report of 1909 to the Royal Commission on the Poor Law, who first proposed a free health service for all: a 'public medical service' or 'state medical service' in her words.

Over the subsequent decades, the Labour party turned that dream into a reality – creating and fighting for a service universal in reach, free at the point of need and forever publicly funded and provided: As Michael Foot told us, it was the greatest socialist achievement of any Labour government.

For me the NHS represents a simple but far reaching and indeed revolutionary ideal, that healthcare should not be an advantage for a privileged few provided by market forces, but the moral right of all. The creation of our National Health Service truly was a civilising moment in our nation's history, as Nye Bevan boasted.

Since 1909, the Fabian Society has remained at the forefront of intellectual debate surrounding the NHS's development. I warmly recall the Fabians' tax commission of 2000, which so influenced that Labour government led by Tony Blair with Gordon Brown as Chancellor – that government showed the political will to increase national insurance, raising billions of pounds for NHS spending. Doing so delivered the lowest waiting times and highest satisfaction rates on record, and it will fall to the next Labour government to restore those standards and provide an ambitious new vision of an NHS which is fit for the future.

I am therefore enormously proud to have curated this collection of essays with the Fabian Society to coincide with the 70th anniversary of our National Health Service, while looking ahead at the future health needs of our population. Our contributors offer provocative insights and, although I suspect the authors won't all agree with one another, a number of themes run throughout all the essays – namely, that a public National Health Service funded through taxation covering all is both the fairest and the most efficient way of providing healthcare.

The condition of the National Health Service in England today with 4 million people on the waiting list, hospitals in perpetual crisis mode, access to primary care frustrated, staff shortages of 100,000 – not to mention the shattering of our social care system – is such that it cries out for a new direction. Labour's commitment is clear: a fully resourced, properly staffed, publicly provided and administered National Health Service alongside a functioning social care service.

Nye Bevan, introducing the NHS in 1948, promised that it would 'lift the shadow from millions of homes'. In her opening essay, Stephanie Snow provides an expert overview of Bevan's vision of a National Health Service, which "rapidly became embedded in British identity". As we plan ahead to the 100th anniversary of the NHS, I believe we must return our NHS to its Bevanite origins – providing the very best healthcare for everyone across society, regardless of their means.

Providing world class healthcare cannot be done on the cheap. Andrew Harrop convincingly outlines the need for substantial additional investment in both the NHS and social care, outlining the damaging consequences of sustained Tory austerity. He persuasively argues we cannot simply rely on productivity gains and hope for the best.

The recent Conservative announcements on spending are a reset from the funding trajectory of the last eight years. But clearly it is not enough investment to deliver the quality of care we need for the future. The government is blatantly conceding that the NHS constitutional standards on waiting times won't be met, risking a middle-class flight as more and more turn to private sector options for elective surgery as waits become too intolerable. What is more, the failure to produce a social care settlement is nothing short of criminal.

An NHS truly fit for the future must also be structured appropriately. Bob Kerslake powerfully argues that the 2012 Health and Social Care Act resulted in a 'fragmented and depleted structure'. The damage understandably stifled any desire from NHS leaders, staff and patients for further structural change, yet we must not shy away from the need for a responsible rethink.

Even Conservative ministers – the same ones who sat in the Cabinet and signed off the Lansley reforms – agree the Health and Social Care Act has created a mess. Labour's clear commitment is to repeal this Act and end privatisation. Over the coming months we want to engage in a debate about how we move to partnership and planning in the delivery of healthcare rather than competition and markets. Lord Kerslake's essay is a welcome and substantial launch of that crucial debate.

And it's a debate that must not be ducked. Labour's ambition to deliver whole person care will demand greater integration, partnership and co-ordination between community care, primary care, mental health services and social care, all working with the acute sector. Of course that means a strategic hand in the planning of healthcare, but Labour cannot endorse new models that allow greater privatisation. The 2012 Act enabled the excesses of the private sector to take hold, to damaging effect for patients and staff. Returning our NHS into public hands is therefore critical, and respected health campaigner John Lister rightly pulls no punches detailing the failures of privatisation in the NHS.

As socialists, our concern is not merely with the equity of the system but the outcomes we want from it too. We should never expect patients to fit to the system of healthcare that is imposed upon them, but always ask how the system of healthcare delivers for the needs of patients. This is why the experience of patients and their families must always be our priority, as Chris Graham rightly argues in his essay.

There is no question that the National Health Service – as that powerful engine of social justice – has led to great advances in life expectancy by offering care for all alongside advances in medicines, treatments and procedures. Living longer and better lives is surely a lodestar we must all be guided by. And yet today gross inequalities still disfigure Britain.

Narrowing health inequalities with a focus on improving the health and wellbeing of every child will be an overarching aim of the next Labour government's health policy, and something I consider my personal mission.

The 1980 Black Report, commissioned by a Labour government, found that in some cases health outcomes were diminishing for the poorest social groups and that the gap between rich and poor had widened. Regrettably, almost four decades on, the findings strike a familiar tone.

Sir Michael Marmot, the world-recognised authority on public health, has warned that since 2010 improvements in life expectancy have stalled, and in some regions worsened. Those from the most deprived backgrounds now enjoy a healthy life expectancy of just 52, which is almost two decades fewer than the least deprived of us.

While we know health outcomes for many conditions have improved nationwide, almost half of the gap in life expectancy between the most and least deprived areas in England is due to excess deaths from heart disease, stroke and cancer in the most deprived areas.

Stark inequalities begin in childhood. Five-year-olds in the most deprived areas are almost seven times more likely to suffer with tooth decay than their peers in the wealthiest areas. The infant mortality rate is more than twice as high in the most deprived areas compared with the least deprived areas.

As Kevin Gulliver powerfully outlines, health inequalities are growing – and they are making the nation sick.

We must consider healthcare treatment not in isolation, but as part of the wider social determinants of health. We know there is a correlation between poverty, deprivation and poor health outcomes.

Lack of access to healthcare in our poorest communities leads to awful consequences. Today we hear of so-called 'DIY dentistry' where those who can't afford dental care are forced to turn to £5 treatments kits from high street discount stores. These kits come with a putty, antiseptic and scraper so those who can't afford it can do their own fillings. Has it really come to this?

A focus on prevention starts from the very beginning of life. Health inequalities are observable from birth – we see it in the low birth rates, mortality rates and breastfeeding rates for those children born in deprivation compared to children from wealthier areas. For too long child health has been neglected as a serious policy priority, storing up substantial problems in later life. For example, the majority of overweight and obese children will remain so in adult life. If the crisis in childhood obesity is not tackled, half of all UK children will be obese or overweight by 2020. Obesity is also twice as common amongst children living in the most deprived areas as compared to children in the most privileged areas.

As Neena Modi powerfully argues: "Child health determines the health of the nation and its prosperity." Labour has proposed radical measures such as restricting the advertising of junk food but we know we must go further too. I have long argued that our children deserve nothing less than being the healthiest children in the world. It is an ambitious target certainly but we must be ambitious for our children. And that involves ensuring fully resourced and timely access to mental health services too for children and adolescents.

Genuine commitment to parity of esteem between mental health and physical health is quite rightly a huge priority for Jeremy Corbyn. For too long mental health has been the Cinderella service of the NHS and yet depression is one of the biggest causes of morbidity in England. As Luciana Berger writes, mental health services have remained 'undervalued and underfunded'. Merely posturing about parity of esteem is not good enough. That is why Labour will substantially increase spending on mental health, and deliver a world-class child and adolescent mental health service.

A modern NHS must also adapt to changing demographics and the nature of ill health in the 21st century. The rising numbers of patients with multiple chronic conditions ongoing care closer to home should be at the very heart of our future strategy. As Paul Williams persuasively argues, if we are to focus 'firmly on prevention', as we must, the role of community care and general practice must be prioritised and properly funded.

Which brings us to the workforce. There are already 100,000 vacancies across the NHS. Estimates suggest in the next 15 years we will need 171,000 extra nurses and 64,000 extra doctors. In social care we will need half a million more staff by 2033/34. We face a workforce crisis and with a projected global shortage of 14.5 million health staff across the world by 2030, alongside Brexit – and with nations like China and India substantially expanding their own health provision – the UK will struggle to recruit internationally in the future in sufficient numbers.

As UNISON's Sara Gorton explains, the number one reason behind public dissatisfaction with the NHS is staffing shortages. Clinical and support staff understandably feel undervalued and underpaid, and yet without their tireless dedication our health service would simply tip over the edge. My aim is that the NHS should be the very best employer in the country. That starts with investing in our NHS staff. We will need a renewed contract of faith with our million-plus NHS staff, who commit their working lives to caring for others and whose care, dedication and self-sacrifice is literally often the difference between life and death.

Since Bevan's creation, healthcare innovation has been nothing short of astonishing. CT and MRI scanners, keyhole surgery, IVF – all have been pioneered in the National Health Service. We are on the cusp of great advances and innovations from additive manufacturing, artificial intelligence, bespoke nutrition and robotics. Digital health technologies are already helping us manage conditions and keep us fit, and it's expected that the internet of things will comprise of 50 trillion devices by the time the NHS reaches its 100th birthday.

No one should fall into the trap of thinking all we need are new exciting gizmos – such an attitude is insulting to staff – but nor should we be luddite in dismissing the potential for healthcare, and crucially public health and prevention, from these technological advances. Tara Donnelly's contribution outlines the remarkable potential of healthcare innovation which, alongside our life sciences sector, has unparalleled potential to improve patient outcomes and increase the wider benefits of the NHS to our economy.

All of us stand proud that Labour's greatest achievement remains so cherished by the public. Our health service is the envy of the world. It is the epitome of compassion in action. But we know we need to go further in the future. The demands of an ageing population require solutions to the social care crisis we are facing but also must surely mean better integration and co-ordination of health and social care delivered at a local level too.

These are all big important questions that require full debate and interrogation. I trust readers will find these essays a useful contribution to that discourse. But while we rightly celebrate 70 years of the NHS this year, we must recognise the dangers ahead and dedicate ourselves to winning the argument again for a properly funded, public National Health Service. It is an argument Labour can win.

1: A SOURCE OF PRIDE: THE NHS AND THE NATION

Stephanie Snow

When it was created, the National Health Service transformed our country. It remains a symbol of compassion, fairness and equality. When we look to reform it, we must ensure we retain the values and principles which have informed it throughout its history.

The 70th anniversary of the National Health Service has generated a wave of celebrations across the UK alongside serious initiatives to address the significant challenges that face today's NHS. Since 1948, NHS history has been characterised by concerns about costs and design, which have prompted successive reforms to resolve these seemingly intractable issues. Within months of its launch, NHS costs exceeded the original estimates of expenditure. Charges were introduced for glasses and dentures in 1951; prescription charges followed in 1952.

The Guillebaud committee was tasked to review the cost of the service in 1953 and published its report in 1956. Contrary to expectations, the committee concluded that the NHS was good value for money and that it justified receiving a greater percentage of the gross national product. It also highlighted the contradictions of the tripartite design of the NHS which brought together hospitals, GPs, dentists, opticians and local authority services.

Since the 1970s, new medical technologies and treatments along with a growing and ageing population have caused governments across the world, particularly those with welfare states and finite budgets, to struggle to provide the best health outcomes. In 2018, concerns about patient safety and effectiveness of care in the NHS are higher than ever, with daily reports of crisis and system failure.

Nevertheless, the anniversary has catalysed an outpouring of support for the institution from staff and patients alike. The NHS is "one of the greatest riches we have as a nation, it is to be treasured, valued and enhanced", one of those we interviewed for our NHS at 70 project told us. To understand the deep and enduring value the NHS holds for people we have to return to its creation and the definitive role of Aneurin Bevan.

Bevan, Wales and the NHS

The NHS that Bevan developed was not a watertight blueprint of services and structures. It brought together a patchwork of existing services and people: more than 3,000 hospitals; more than 250,000 staff and 1000s of GP practices and public health services. Opposition to its creation came from all quarters; doctors who did not want to become instruments of the state; MPs who feared the economic and social burden for the state; local authorities which resisted losing control of their hospitals; and teaching hospitals wanting to preserve their independence. "The new Health Service has been having a most uneasy gestation and a very turbulent birth, but all prodigies behave like that," Bevan said on 25 June 1948. The glue that stuck the NHS together and has kept it at the centre of British everyday life over the past 70 years was Bevan's vision of improving health by establishing free and equal access to care determined by clinical need rather than ability to pay.

From the 1900s onwards, ideas of a comprehensive health system had emerged in Britain from various quarters including the Fabian Society. By the second world war, there was a broad consensus around the need for a collective system although assumptions were that such a system would develop from established structures including local authorities and voluntary hospitals and be financed through health insurance. The Labour party's landslide election victory in 1945 was unexpected and resulted in Bevan becoming a minister in Clement Attlee's government. In its form and spirit, the service that was launched on 5 July 1948 was the product of its creator.

Bevan was born in 1897 in Tredegar, a mining town in the South Wales valleys. His father was a miner, his mother a seamstress, and Bevan left school at the age of 13 to work in the colliery. He saw his friends struggle through the Great Depression, some emigrating to find new opportunities. He became involved in trades unions and local politics and led local miners in the general strike of 1926. In 1929, the year of the stock market crash, Bevan was elected as MP for Ebbw Vale. Bevan's political activities, at local and national level, were rooted in his experiences of living and working in the South Wales valleys where the physical and intellectual landscape was carved out by the mining and steel industries and working class struggles for better wages and working conditions. Tredegar was notable for having a Workmen's Medical Aid Society which had been formed in 1890 and by 1933 supplied 95 per cent of the local population's health needs. Philip Prosser, born in 1939 with 'club foot', was able to have several surgical operations because his father paid a weekly subscription to the society. "It was exactly the same as the NHS in 1948. We already had it in Tredegar before that," he said in an NHS at 70 interview.

Close connections between Bevan's early experiences and his development of the NHS are revealed in his collection of essays, In Place of Fear, published in 1952. These illuminate his belief in the need for the welfare of 'ordinary men and women' to be placed high on the political agenda and explain how his political activities were shaped by the 'texture' of his life as a young miner. In a chapter entitled A Free Health Service, Bevan discusses the principles which informed the NHS; that medical treatment and care is a collective responsibility and should be made available to people regardless of ability to pay, according to medical need and no other criteria. Financial anxiety during sickness hindered recovery and was unnecessarily cruel, he insisted. The fear of heavy medical bills caused people to delay seeking medical attention which resulted in more sickness and often permanent disability. He highlighted the particular needs of mothers who suffered most from lack of free healthcare because 'she puts her own needs last'. Financing the health service out of general taxation was, he argued, a much fairer way of ensuring that all citizens had equal access to care when they were sick.

Bevan's vision of a universal health service, free at the point of need, disrupted earlier ideas but it chimed strongly with the post-war public appetite for establishing a fairer society and a new social order. It was rooted in Bevan's deep understanding of the centrality of health for individuals, communities and social productivity and it attracted people like Joan Meredith to campaign for a national health service.

"We just wanted one that was free you know. That everybody could have... I belonged to an organisation – the Young Christian Workers – that did want to help people, that did do that through politics... because we wanted to change the world, we wanted to have some kind of equality and particularly for poor people," she said in her NHS at 70 interview.

The NHS and British identity

The NHS became rapidly embedded in British identity. The service was "a notable exhibit in the shop-window of our British way of life", noted Teddy Chester, director of the Acton Trust, in 1955. By the late 1950s, it was difficult for 'the average Englishman' to imagine life without a health service as it had 'contributed so much to his physical and mental well-being', observed Almont Lindsay, professor of history at the University of Virginia. Bevan was sanguine about the defects in the service such as the continuing existence of pay beds in hospitals and anticipated the need for improvements on every level. His pride lay in the 'massive contribution' the NHS was making 'to the equipment of a civilised society'. He added: "It has now become part of the texture of our national life."

Throughout its 70 years, the NHS has retained its prominence in British life. This was demonstrated in 2012, when frilly-capped nurses and doctors (many of them NHS staff) danced around hospital beds in the extravaganza that opened the London Olympic Games. It was a 'quintessentially British spectacle', observed American commentator, Cassie Chambers. For US citizens, healthcare systems and national pride were not natural bedfellows, but Chambers said she was transfixed by the use of the NHS as a symbol of achievement and inspired by seeing the 'UK vision on display'.

NHS at 70 has been collecting interviews from patients and staff ranging in age from 18 to 97 years. Those in their 80s and 90s who witnessed the beginning of the NHS have nuanced memories. Families who could afford to pay for medical care and those covered by subscription schemes noticed little difference. For poorer people, it transformed lives, entitling them to treatment they had not previously been able to afford. Across the generations people have shared their experiences of poor quality care, disillusionment with political reforms, racial discrimination and the stress of working and being treated in an overloaded system. They advocate the need for change on many levels, they talk about using private medicine to circumvent long waiting lists or travelling abroad for better quality treatment. Nevertheless, their pride and belief in NHS principles remain steadfast. The NHS is synonymous with freedom from the fear of the consequences of ill-health for individuals and their families. When asked what value the NHS holds for them, many people reply simply: "I owe it my life."

For staff, sharing the most difficult parts of people's lives leaves an emotional legacy. A retired nurse told us that 40 years on, she still remembered the names of children who had died on her ward. Interviewees also have a strong awareness, and sometimes direct experience, of what life is like in other countries where access to healthcare can be limited by financial means. For this reason, the NHS is seen as a source of national pride and described by some as 'the envy of the world'.

Going forward

Understanding the enduring value the NHS has for people, whatever the everyday deficiencies in services, is essential for policy makers considering reform. People remain committed to the idea of an NHS because it is a symbol of compassion, fairness and equality. It is woven so tightly into the fabric of their everyday lives, from conception through to death, that contemplating its disappearance or significant alteration is unimaginable. For this reason, public resistance to hospital closures and reorganisation of services that appear to diminish access to care has been extremely strong over the course of NHS history. For many people, the NHS is the 'still point of a turning world' and it is no coincidence that the 70th anniversary is generating so much support given the wider context of Brexit and fractured views about the UK's identity and place in the world.

After Bevan's death in 1960, Jennie Lee, his wife, wrote: "He was a great humanist whose religion lay in loving his fellow men and trying to serve them." The NHS grew out of Bevan's vision to improve life and limit suffering for all members of society and it continues, however imperfectly, to encapsulate these values for people. Seventy years after its creation it stands as the strongest benchmark of humanitarianism and civilisation in UK life.

NHS at 70: The Story of Our Lives is a national programme of work, supported by the Heritage Lottery Fund and led from the University of Manchester, training volunteers to collect stories from patients, staff and the public to capture the place of the NHS in everyday life since 1948. www.nhs70.org.uk

2: STARTING YOUNG: ENSURING HEALTHY CHILDHOODS AND HEALTHY LIVES

Neena Modi

Child health determines the health of the nation – and its prosperity. Preventing ill-health from an early age should therefore be the key focus for government. We need a new Nye Bevan with the vision to make this a reality.

Child health in the UK today is not as good as it should be. A fifth of five-year-olds and a third of 10-year-olds are overweight or obese, for example. One in three five-year-old children have dental caries, an entirely preventable condition, and admissions and deaths for asthma are higher than in many comparable European countries.

Child health is not just important for children. Child health is also a powerful determinant of adult health, population health and national prosperity. For example, the majority of overweight and obese children will remain so in adult life. Obesity will shorten their lifespans and lead to the loss of between 15 and 20 years of healthy adult life. Their risks of developing type 2 diabetes, hypertension, and heart disease will be increased. They will add to the growing prevalence of chronic, non-communicable diseases that are crippling economies and health systems worldwide, and that has led, for the first time in history, to a reduction in America, over the last two consecutive years, of the life span of adults.

The NHS and child health

In all too many parts of the world today, and in the UK prior to 1948, healthcare was built around insurance, out-of-pocket payments, and charity. Children, particularly the children of the unemployed or poor, fared worst of all. The coming of the NHS brought an incalculable change; since its inception, no parent in Britain has had to live with the fear of not being able to afford healthcare for a sick child.

The NHS is a powerful concept – healthcare for all, free at the point of need, funded through general taxation, available to all according to need, not ability to pay. It is magnificent in its simplicity, humanity, and wisdom. Beveridge's aspiration was for 'a national health service for prevention and comprehensive treatment', but in the 1948 articulation of the NHS, the focus was predominantly on healthcare, not health, with the assumption that the predominant determinant of the latter is the former. Today, 70 years later, science shows clearly the extent to which health is the product of far more than healthcare.

What determines health?

Our health trajectories are initiated early, starting when our parent's sperm and eggs are formed, then progressively influenced by the intrauterine environment, the postnatal environment and exposures in childhood and adult life. Injuries and accidents apart, health is the result of external factors interacting with our genes to determine how the messages they hold are translated. We have control over some, but not all, of these factors.

Child health is influenced by conditions in early development and in turn influences health in adult life. Our health as adults, affects the health of our children. If your mother, and possibly your father, were overweight, or malnourished, your risk of developing diabetes in adult life is substantially increased. If your mother smoked during pregnancy, you are at greater risk of chronic respiratory disease in old age, even though you seemed well in early adult life. And if as you grow older, you eat too much, live a sedentary life, and are exposed to air pollution or environmental toxins, further risks are added to a trajectory that leads to poor health in old age.

Advocacy for child health

Advocacy for child health has traditionally focused upon the moral case, though there is a very powerful scientific and economic case as well. Why then isn't there a greater drive to improve child health? Is it because advocacy on behalf of children has been insufficiently persuasive? Is it because the wider long-term benefits to the nation are insufficiently understood? Is it that treatment not prevention is the predominant driver of healthcare systems in the UK and around the world? Is it that political ability to define the actions that are needed, and the will to implement change are lacking? Or is it that children have no vote and no voice and therefore their perspectives remain unheard by governments and outweighed by mighty corporations?

Dangers for child health ahead

Although a primarily publicly funded, delivered, and accountable healthcare system is the most effective means of reducing both healthcare costs and demand, we are witnessing the introduction in the UK of an ideology which is particularly damaging to children. In this ideology, health is a matter of personal choice and healthcare is a commodity where activity and profit – not health – are the metrics of success. Here, it is argued, if an adult chooses to smoke and as a consequence gets cancer, let him pay for treatment, just as he pays for housing, food and clothing. Even if he didn't smoke and the cancer was no fault of his, he should have the sense to insure himself against such misfortune, rather than expecting the bill to be picked up by the taxpayer.

Children cannot exercise personal choice, and further, they stand to benefit the most from preventive measures. The view that there is benefit in treating healthcare as a commodity is particularly damaging to children because prevention can't readily be bought and sold, unlike treatments. Thus in a marketised model, industries that thrive on ill health are promoted, be they insurers, for-profit providers, or the manufacturers of diagnostics and pharmaceuticals. Additionally, when health is considered primarily a matter of personal choice, industries that cause poor health also prosper. The long drawn-out battles to curb the powers of the tobacco, alcohol and junk food industries are cases in point. Health gains have been delayed with unquantifiable damage to children – and ultimately to the adult population – by superficial arguments that these industries boost the economy, raise tax revenues, and create jobs.

Proponents of a marketised model argue that care for needy children can be provided by charity, as with the large US children's hospitals, or by a supposedly benevolent state that picks up on payments. However, a need for charity is a cardinal expression of inequity in society, and state provision of healthcare for children is no redress against poor preventive health policies.

The current system

The current NHS doesn't have responsibility for health, only for shouldering the consequences. The NHS can deal with illness and injury, but whose responsibility is it to address the early developmental and wider societal conditions that lead to ill-health or disease? Take the example of smoking, unequivocally shown to be bad for the health of those who smoke, their children, and those around them. Public information and education campaigns sustained over several decades made insufficient impact on reducing smoking prevalence. The measures that worked were the ban on public smoking (a public health measure), plain packaging (a regulatory measure), and increased taxation (a fiscal measure). Sadly, no cabinet minister today has responsibility for ensuring that national policies do not adversely impact upon health. Additionally, public health budgets are devolved to local authorities, an unnecessary abrogation of central responsibility given that the UK is a small country with relatively homogenous conditions and populations. Devolving responsibility for public health, with a repetitive review of evidence by each local authority, and decision-making criteria that differ around the country, is wasteful and inefficient. It is not surprising that the result is a post-code lottery where what is delivered comes down to the luck of the draw. The population would be far better served if evidence were reviewed and decisions made centrally and policies were applied consistently.

The current discourse about the NHS scratches the surface, and does not get to the root cause of the prevailing malaise. The NHS as a cohesive entity no longer exists. The current UK healthcare system is fragmented – across the four nations, within England, and between public health, primary care, hospital and community services. Responsibility for training healthcare professionals is divorced from responsibility for provision of care and from immigration rulings regarding overseas staff. It is increasingly inefficient, as a confusing mix of public sector, private, and social enterprise providers are awarded public funds to deliver to contract, not to deliver health. It is unclear where responsibility now lies, as evidenced by the extraordinary spectacle of the non-elected chief executive of NHS England calling for more funding while government dissociates itself from responsibility.

Wilfully or out of ignorance, as all evidence points to the contrary, false mantras are being promulgated, that universal healthcare is unaffordable and that a dominant private sector can deliver more efficiently than the public sector. The costs of healthcare are exorbitant only in inefficient systems. The NHS is the most cost-effective healthcare system that has ever existed and the UK pioneered the underpinning principles of the National Institute for Health and Care Excellence, namely fair cost containment based upon evidence. An exclusively or predominantly private system, in which a patient buys (directly or indirectly) and a doctor (or healthcare provider organisation) sells, or a system that is publicly funded but not publicly delivered as is increasingly the case in England, is multiply damaging. Administrative costs and charges upon the taxpayer are increased. Perverse incentives are introduced and trust between doctor and patient is compromised. When money is the driving force for healthcare, everyone suffers; the poor from lack of care, the rich from over-investigation and anxiety, and preventive health takes second place.

A better future

More funding for UK health services is certainly needed, but in large part, this is a distraction. So too is the endless reworking of so-called models of care. UK healthcare – for which read the NHS – needs to be brought conceptually into 21st century thinking.

In a better system, health would be the desired outcome, not healthcare. Preventive health, focusing on early development and childhood, would be a cardinal focus. There would be clear understanding of the implications of the science of the early developmental origins and wider determinants of health and disease. These insights would be translated into policies underpinned by recognition of the national benefit that would result from adopting 'life-course' and 'health in all policies' approaches to health. The life-course approach would be operationalised by bringing public and preventive health together with primary, acute and long-term care, under the banner of the NHS. A 'health in all policies' approach would mean that the health impact of policies would be a prime consideration for their adoption. The increasingly and unnecessarily fragmented funding and provider structure would be replaced with a system that is predominantly publicly delivered, integrated, and evaluated against nationally consistent criteria relevant to health, not to process, activity or profit. Private sector involvement in healthcare would be limited. Equitable cost containment methodologies would be improved, and coupled with fair assessment of what the nation could afford. Cabinet level responsibility and accountability for the quality and availability of healthcare would be reintroduced. The healthcare workforce would be valued and sustained, with an expansion in numbers, the return of nationally consistent terms and conditions, and a secure pension. And lowering the voting age, and possibly too, issuing parents with a proxy vote for each underage child would focus political minds upon policies that benefit children.

Such change would no doubt be fiercely contested, just as was the introduction of the NHS. The country needs a Nye Bevan of the 21st century, a politician who understands that enriching the founding principles of the NHS with insights from science offers the opportunity to leave a lasting positive legacy for the nation, and who has the commitment and ability to carry through such visionary change.

3: AN EQUAL STAKE?:
TACKLING HEALTH INEQUALITIES

Kevin Gulliver

Economic inequalities are stark and increasing and they are making the nation sick. If people's health is no longer to be defined by where they were born, then we must put tackling these inequalities in life chances, income and housing at the heart of a national strategy.

In this, the 70th anniversary year of the National Health Service, healthcare delivery and funding are at the top of the domestic political agenda. But while the NHS remains one of the most cherished of the UK's institutions, the erosion of health funding as a proportion of gross domestic product has been accompanied by a slump in public satisfaction of 13 per cent since 2010. Even with the promised new funding announced by prime minister Theresa May, real terms spending on the NHS will only have returned to 2010 levels by 2024. Dwindling expenditure over the last eight years has precipitated a series of winter crises, ongoing strain on A&E departments, and haemorrhaging of NHS staff – exacerbated by Brexit and pay freezes. For the first time since statistics were first assembled, improvements in life expectancy in the UK have stalled – especially in the poorest areas – with austerity policy enacted from 2010 a key driver.

As public health professionals have recorded for some considerable time – although their collective voice has been diminished as the public health service has been reorganised and denuded – access to good quality healthcare is only one of the factors in determining how long we live and our freedom from sickness as a prerequisite of a good quality of life. Lifestyle and socio-economic characteristics, as well as geographical inequities in access to healthcare, are key contributors to life expectancy and illness rates. Even though the NHS has been central in improving both health and wellbeing over seven decades, health inequalities exist and persist. These inequalities cannot be explained only by differentials in access to healthcare. Not all citizens have an equal stake in the nation's healthcare system; not least because delivering equal health outcomes is beyond any healthcare system. If health inequalities are to be tackled, then we must look at the circumstances of people's lives, their social status, the economic disparities they face and where they live and their housing needs

Growing inequality, poverty and destitution

The UK is one of the most unequal among the world's industrialised nations, and has seen a rapid growth in poverty and destitution since the financial crash of 2007/08. According to the Equality Trust, the UK's wealth divide has widened considerably since 2010. Just 1,000 individuals have amassed a total wealth of £724bn, including property, pensions, investments and possessions, which is significantly greater than that of the poorest 40 per cent of households, who have a combined wealth of just £567bn. Just 20 individuals control assets of £192bn, or 1.5 per cent of UK wealth. The UK's 1,000 richest people have increased their wealth by £66bn in the past year alone, and by £274bn in the past five years; an increase of 61 per cent over half a decade and equivalent to more than two years' spending on the NHS.

In 2017, 14.3m people were in relative poverty in the UK – up 300,000 from the previous year. Of these, 4.1m were children. Poverty is set to rise sharply in the next three years as tax and benefit changes, enacted since 2010, begin to bite. The Institute of Fiscal Studies calculates that those in the lowest income deciles will see a fall in their real terms incomes of up to 10 per cent while more affluent households will stay about the same or see a small rise. At the sharp end of the income spectrum, 1.5m people in the UK were classified as destitute by the Joseph Rowntree Foundation. And the use of food banks has escalated from 41,000 to more than 2 million since 2010, driven by muddled implementation of universal credit, the introduction of the bedroom tax, and punitive welfare benefit sanctions. These increases in economic inequality, in poverty and destitution, all have profound implications for health inequities.

Health inequalities and the 'social determinants'

A deep and wide body of evidence, stretching back at least 30 years, reveals disparities in mortality and morbidity rates in the UK. Health inequalities are largely a reflection of socio-economic inequalities embedded in the national fabric. The Marmot Review of 2010 – Fair Society, Healthy Lives – commented that social and economic differences in health status reflect, and are caused by, social and economic inequalities in society. Unequal access to resources – money, power, knowledge, prestige and beneficial social networks – has consequence for health status. Poorer people have shorter, sicker lives, while the more affluent are able to avoid health risks, disease, and the consequences of disease. Health inequalities have also been recorded between men and women, ethnic groups, neighbourhoods and tenure.

The 'social determinants' of health match the distribution of economic and social conditions among the population. Class, relative wealth and poverty, and the perceptions that different class groupings have of their relative status in society, are all arranged on a 'social gradient' running from top to bottom of the economy and society, with 'high' status individuals having better health than those of 'low' status. Increasing levels of poor health appear on every rung of the ladder going down from top to bottom. The distribution of social determinants is shaped by a range of factors: prevailing economic and political ideologies, public policy-making, the universality of welfare and prevailing levels of inequality within countries. Unfair economic outcomes, poor or inadequate social policies, and a growing gap between rich and poor, all affect how long we live and the quality of our health.

The power of place

The role of geography in determining how long we live and our comparative health and wellbeing is increasingly recognised. 'Place' is an important determinant of health status, above and beyond the clustering of disadvantaged or affluent groups in discernible neighbourhoods. A number of acknowledged neighbourhood effects, such as population density, relative air quality and concentrations of poor housing, all have an impact on health and wellbeing. There is also a strong relationship between deprivation levels and life expectancy and illness rates. Those living in the bottom fifth most deprived neighbourhoods have a life expectancy at birth of almost a decade below people living in the most affluent fifth. The life expectancy gap is even starker between the very poorest neighbourhoods and the super-affluent, ranging from 15 to 18 years. Conclusion: neighbourhood deprivation means shorter, sicker lives for residents.

Health and housing

Health fissures have opened up because of a doubling of homelessness, rough sleeping, and use of temporary housing in the last eight years. The main reason for becoming homeless is eviction from the insecure private rented sector, a sector which has doubled in size over the last two decades. The average life expectancy of a rough sleeper is just 47 years for a man and 43 years for a woman. There are almost 1.2m households on local council waiting lists, and the government's own figures point to a need for 300,000 new homes annually to clear the backlog of housing needs and to meet the demand from newly forming households.

Poor and overcrowded housing poses major risks to health, including poor mental health, respiratory disease, long-term health and disability and the delayed physical and cognitive development of children. Cold housing is especially damaging for health and causes an estimated fifth of excess winter deaths, and insecure and short-term tenure housing is damaging for physical and mental health. Much of the country's worst housing is located in the poorest neighbourhoods. Levels of poor, hazardous and overcrowded housing are on the rise. It is estimated by the Building Research Establishment that poor housing costs the NHS £1.4bn annually.

An equal stake – tackling health inequalities

To ensure that all UK citizens have an equal stake in the NHS, we will have to spend more. We will need to focus on eradicating the health inequalities which exist because of unequal access to services, eliminating of the postcode lottery, and bolstering public health services at the local level. But it's not just about money for health services: we need to create and implement a national strategy to reduce economic inequalities, poverty and destitution. Such a strategy needs to target income and wealth inequalities, to raise wages and benefits, and to extend asset ownership to ensure a more equitable share of national resources. Most importantly, policies that bear down on poverty, especially child poverty, such as introduction of a real living wage, a more generous social security system for working age people, and approaches to redistributing income and wealth through the tax system, must be at the heart of the strategy. A universal basic income, the creation of sovereign wealth funds, and more localised and mutualised economies in urban and rural settings might all be considered as part of this approach.

Localised and community-centred initiatives should be developed and/or reinvigorated alongside national fiscal and welfare actions. Drastic cuts in local government and social housing budgets should be reversed to improve the life chances, housing and neighbourhood conditions of disadvantaged communities. The rejuvenation of Sure Start centres, advice services and community facilities would foster more resilient communities and bolster community self-esteem. Our research[1] shows how the Black County Housing Group in Dudley and Sandwell is achieving high levels of community investment to improve the financial circumstances, health and wellbeing of residents. Nehemiah UCHA – a BME housing association – offers services that improve wellbeing and reduce loneliness. Accord's Holiday Kitchen in Birmingham provides family wellbeing support and healthy communal meals for pre and primary aged children during school holidays. And People's Health Trust enables 'local conversations' to confront health inequalities in some of the country's most deprived communities. These initiatives have helped improve the health and wellbeing of local people, and boosted self-esteem, but can only become embedded in the long-term if the macro-economic environment moves towards greater equality.

Of course, implementing an overarching plan to ensure a more equal UK does not come cheap. A more progressive income tax system would be a good starting pointing to fund the strategy. The introduction of a wealth tax on the richest segment of society, who have seen their assets growth exponentially as others have faced wage stagnation, could yield significant sums. Scoping a land value tax, and reshaping council tax bands, would also make a fairer Britain while tackling underfunding of local government and resolving the housing crisis. The scale of the endeavour will need to be ambitious, but investment in greater equality will save money for the NHS – and create a healthier Britain.

4: STRUCTURAL ISSUES: CREATING AN NHS THAT WORKS BETTER

Bob Kerslake

The last major overhaul of NHS structures in 2012 was so brutal that many said 'never again'. But the time is now right for better planned and more inclusive reforms to put NHS providers on a more sustainable footing and leave the health service as a whole well-placed for the future.

Much has been written about the funding issues facing the NHS at 70. Much less has been said about reforming NHS structures.

This is the correct order of things. Organisations can generally get by with poor structures if the finances are sound. However no organisation, no matter how brilliant, can function properly with the scale of funding crisis currently facing the NHS. I am pleased and relieved that the long period of denial of this reality might just be coming to an end.

If we want to create an NHS that is truly sustainable for the future, however, we do need to look again at how it is organised. What we have now is palpably not fit for purpose.

The 2010 coalition government quickly established a programme of ambitious reform across pretty much the whole of the public sector. This was in part driven by austerity but also by the pent-up ambitions of ministers achieving office after a long period in opposition. At the same time, David Cameron significantly reduced the capacity at the centre of government to review and scrutinise what was coming forward from departments.

This 'fast and furious' approach to reform brought with it significant problems across government, for example the well-publicised difficulties with universal credit. But by far and away the biggest difficulties came in the reforms brought in by the Health and Social Care Act 2012. The process of change was disruptive enough. It is a testimony to the work of senior leaders such as former NHS England chief executive David Nicholson that the wheels didn't come off completely. However, much more serious was what was left after the dust had settled. A fragmented and depleted structure had been created that was singularly ill-equipped to meet the future needs of the service.

By the end of the coalition government there were two prevailing conclusions about the reforms. First, that they have been a missed opportunity at best and a disaster at worst. Second, that the upheaval and general grief caused by the reorganisation meant that there could be no prospect of further organisational change.

The result of this view, carried forward in to the 2015 government and Theresa May's administration that followed it, has meant that subesequent reorganisation has happened by stealth. Some of this change has not been without merit, for example the creation of sustainability and transformation partnerships and the establishment of integrated care systems have promoted wider collaboration. Bringing together clinical commissioning groups in some areas has reduced costs. However the overall effect has been piecemeal and lacking in coherence. The absence of a clearly articulated plan has led some to raise issues of accountability and question whether there is a hidden agenda.

We are now six years on from the Lansley reforms. If the next general election happens to schedule in 2022, we will be a decade on from them. Enough time has now passed to contemplate further organisational change to put the deficiencies right.

What changes might be needed? First, it is important to say that the way the organisations of the NHS have worked has been significantly influenced by the funding crisis. NHS Improvement, for example – notwithstanding the brave vision of its first chair Ed Smith – has become 'NHS Containment' or 'NHS Enforcement', acting on behalf of the secretary of state to bear down on provider finance and performance.

It is worth stepping outside of the world of the NHS to see just how different things are. In the worlds of housing associations, universities, schools and local government, all areas that I have some knowledge of, there are certainly differences in performance and financial strength between different institutions. There are also financial challenges and uncertainties for the future. However the prevailing norm is of sustainable and viable organisations. Intervention by the regulator or government is the absolute exception. In the case of local government, for example, despite the swingeing cuts in funding that councils have experienced since 2010, the number of interventions can be counted on one hand and only one of these was for financial reasons.

Much has been said about getting 'more from more' if additional NHS funding is provided. However the most essential task that must be taken first is to 'reset' the NHS and put its providers on a path to the sustainability that is taken for granted in other sectors. Accumulated deficits need to be addressed and working balances established. Funding needs to be adequate to realistically set balanced budgets and deliver the expected performance standards. The tariff funding model needs radical overhaul to make it simpler and more predictable.

Achieving this would allow a significant simplification of the national structures, lower costs and a reduction in the conflicting and duplicated demands for information from providers. As with other sectors, such as housing, there should be a single commissioner in NHS England and a single regulator combining CQC and the regulatory role of NHSI covering quality, governance and financial viability.[2] Further simplification and cost reduction could be achieved by reviewing whether we need to retain Public Health England and Health Education England as freestanding organisations. The regional structures of NHSE should be strengthened and aligned to the emerging economic 'meta regions' of the North, the Midlands, the South West, London and the South East.[3]

If the reset has been done properly, there should then be space for the Department of Health, the national commissioner and regulator to spend less time on fire fighting and more on exploring the longer term strategic issues. In particular, there is an urgent need for a proper investment plan for buildings and technology linked to a vision of how the NHS will work in the future. We have ended the PFI programme but not replaced it with a credible, funded plan for long-term investment.

At local level, it is equally important to fix the funding of social care. Without addressing this growing funding gap, the future viability of local government is in doubt and it will certainly not be able to play its part in developing joint systems of health and care. There is a real fear in local government that any extra funding will only be for the NHS and meeting the needs of social care will be pushed off to a later date. This would be a grave mistake on the part of the government. In some parts of the country, the private social care market is close to collapse.

Assuming that social care funding will be addressed, there is a real opportunity to develop new devolved local commissioning models building on the example created in Greater Manchester. The arrangements will vary across the country reflecting local needs, but need to be guided by a clear set of organising principles. Greater local government engagement and indeed leadership of merged arrangements would strengthen accountability and reduce some of the concerns that have developed about 'creeping privatisation'.

A huge simplification and reduction in costly bureaucracy could be achieved by moving away from the current commissioner provider split at local level and introducing long term 10-year contracts based on the size and needs of the local population. More of the NHS commissioning budget, for example for mental health services, could be determined locally. There should be the opportunity to reconfigure clinical commissioning group boundaries to better align with those of local government.

Tempting though it might be to some, I would not advocate taking social care funding out of local government. It is too entangled with the wider funding changes in local government, in particular the planned full retention of business rates, and would represent a major reversal of the devolution agenda. Much can be achieved through greater flexibility and alignment of funds at local level.

Improving public health is critical to managing the future demands on the NHS. One of the good things in the 2012 Act was that it passed responsibility for the public health function to local government. It has much better access to the leavers needed to improve fitness and tackle obesity. However, for funding or other reasons, this change has not yet had the impact originally hoped for and there is a case for looking again at the organisational arrangements.

Finally, as part of freeing up decision-making at local level, the 'any willing provider' provision in the 2012 Act should be removed. It is likely that a mixed market of provision involving the private and independent sector will need to continue, if only to deal with peaks in demand. However there should be more local discretion on what to buy externally and who to buy it from.

Structural change always brings with it additional uncertainty and cost. It should not therefore be entered into lightly. It would almost certainly require new primary legislation. However I think it is time to recognise that the problems created by the 2012 Act cannot be fully addressed without this. Change does not need to be done in the top-down, brutal way that has often characterised previous NHS restructurings. There is scope for a better planned and more inclusive approach. It can and must be achieved without any adverse impact on patient care.

There is little doubt in my mind though that change is needed.

5: PUTTING THE NHS IN OUR POCKETS: THE ROLE OF DIGITAL INNOVATION

Tara Donnelly

The NHS has always innovated – so where should it be looking to go next in the years to come? Digital innovation is not a panacea, but it's the most distinct opportunity in healthcare right now. It could being new solutions to old problems if it is done on the right scale.

I started working in the NHS in 1988, as a ward house-keeper in a busy coronary care ward. My early days were about playing my part in the ward team; directly helping patients, their relatives and clinical staff. It was incredibly rewarding, and was why I decided to return to the NHS after university to build a career here, a decision I've never regretted. After a range of clinical management roles I worked my way up to executive level positions, ran a hospital in west London and now lead an organisation dedicated to helping the NHS improve and make the most of innovations; we call it 'speeding up the best'.

During that 30-year period though, there were of course ups and downs. But I can also say this: there was not a day where I doubted the innovative spirit of the NHS. The evidence is clear – in its first 70 years the NHS has been responsible for innovations that have changed healthcare around the world. The first MRI scanner, the first CT scanner, the health system to pioneer IVF. Let's not forget that the NHS itself is one of the world's greatest innovations and it's an innovation that treats one million people every 36 hours, with the vast majority of those people receiving safe, compassionate care, free at the point of use.

I vividly remember witnessing the extraordinary impact of clot-busting drugs in stroke care. I used to make a point of regularly visiting the stroke ward at the hospital I ran, because they were tough places to be and work. Patients were visibly affected and stricken, relatives often weeping, it was extraordinary how staff managed to remain both cheerful and compassionate. You walk onto a hyper-acute stroke ward now and it is though a miracle has occurred; some of the patients are laughing, joking and walking around the ward the day after having a major stroke. This is the impact of innovation in technology combined with innovation in service design – in this case getting people to centres where they can have their brain imaged and clotbusters given within hours of a 'brain attack' which massively reduces the damage to many people, and is saving many lives daily.

As the NHS marks its 70th year, the need to unleash this spirit and innovate faster and further is undisputed. We know our population is ageing, we know that people are increasingly developing multiple long-term conditions that require time and resource from the NHS. We know that more of the same simply will not do.

Digital solutions to old problems

Technology and innovation are not a panacea to these problems, but I believe passionately that they can help address them. When we bank, travel, order food – we do it digitally. When we interact with the NHS, we rarely do. When we bank, travel, order food – the solution is in our pocket. When we think about our health, we use our smartphone only to call someone, and then dutifully wait to receive our appointments by letter.

Taking appointments as an example: many, many trees are felled and the NHS remains the biggest user of second class mail in the world, spending approximately £20m a year on postage. The majority of this is spent sending letters to advise on clinic times. Things are starting to change, however, with solutions like DrDoctor, a smartphone-based digital outpatients platform. In my patch, we've already seen huge benefits from this kind of digital approach. Guy's and St Thomas' NHS Foundation Trust provides well over a million clinic appointments each year and it uses the product across all of them because it gives patients much more say in selecting a date and time of their choice, resulting in 'no show' rates falling by around 40 per cent. The feedback from patients is incredibly positive, it reduces waiting times by three weeks typically, plus it saves the hospital a much needed £3m a year.

Beyond outpatient services, there are other digital solutions leading a quiet revolution in some aspects of clinical care. One example is in care for chronic obstructive pulmonary disease (COPD), the umbrella term for a range of relatively common progressive lung diseases including emphysema, chronic bronchitis, and refractory asthma. Respiratory disease, including the COPD group, is the second most common reason for emergency hospital admission in this country, and it is highly seasonal. It is also much more common in people who are vulnerable and are deprived or in lower social economic groups. The better news is that while COPD is a chronic lifelong and worsening condition, it is highly amenable and responsive to self-management.

An entrepreneurial British respiratory physician called Simon Bourne developed a digital platform called myCOPD that covers all aspects of managing the condition. It uses the behavioural insights knowledge combined with great technology to make high quality self-management possible. By using the platform regularly to complete rehabilitation exercises, and correct their inhaler technique, people are able to keep themselves well for much longer, and reduce exacerbations that bring them into hospital. We now have 50,000 people using this solution, across the NHS.

Spreading innovation at scale

myCOPD is part of a small group of digital health solutions achieving such stunning results that they are matching and in some cases surpassing the impact of medication, treatment, therapy and consultations; we call them 'digital therapeutics'.

Recent analysis from health technology company IQVIA demonstrates that if we were to systematically implement those digital solutions with the strongest evidence base in just five clinical areas the impact on patients would be phenomenal. Results would include powerful change effects in terms of weight loss, stability of blood glucose levels, increased activity including undertaking regular exercise as part of cardiac and pulmonary rehabilitation, reduced breathlessness, better adherence to medicine, improved inhaler technique, fewer GP and hospital visits.

In addition to the clinical and patient benefits, their analysis finds that the savings from implementing across five conditions alone would be £170m recurrent each year, much of this in much-needed clinical time.

Barriers to spread

The need to spread digital therapeutics and other technological advances across the NHS is obvious, and progress is being made. But it is slower than it should be. If we accept that the NHS is innovative at its core, what are the barriers?

We're currently working with a number of hospitals and a mental health service across London who are looking to digitise the way they communicate and operate their outpatient services. Their take on the barriers is stark. It's not the age-old idea that clinicians aren't up for change. Clinicians want new solutions that will help their patients and free up their time. Neither is it a lack of patient demand – patients want new ways of managing their conditions and interacting with the health service. It is the system that they are operating in and a lack of resource to implement new solutions.

The most common issue we hear of is the tariff, the way the NHS is paid for activity. It includes perverse disincentives to digital, as on the national tariff trusts are paid a fraction of what they are paid for a face-to-face, if they offer the consultation 'virtually'. This is despite the feedback from large cohorts of patients that this is their preferred way of seeing their clinician.

It is also time and resource. The NHS spends 0.035 per cent of its budget on dedicated activity to 'spread' its innovations. When we look at those private sector companies with an innovation focus, whether in tech or drug development, they all spend two to three times what they spend in research and development on their spread effort, in their case sales and marketing. In the NHS we spend under 5 per cent of our research spend on dedicated spread activity. If we matched the ratios the private sector use, rather than spending £44m a year, it would be £3bn.

Being bold

As the NHS turns 70, we have an opportunity to be bold with digital. We can invest in digital therapeutics at scale. Starting with the five areas the IQVIA study examines: prediabetes, diabetes, COPD, cardiac rehab and asthma, we have a real chance to make mainstream what is currently novel. We should create a digital innovation fund to support those parts of the NHS keen to make the most of digital opportunities do so and at rapid pace.

We need to be bold with devices too. Not all parts of the population can access digital solutions. But that's not the same as saying that they couldn't benefit, if access were improved. There's good evidence that digitally excluded groups, including the homeless and parts of the prison population, could radically improve their health with a smartphone or telemedicine. Why not find ways to give more devices to those who benefit most, either through recycling schemes, or even a private sector funded NHS birthday present of devices for healthcare use?

The sooner we can get securely held patient records and results into the hands of activated and educated patients the better. There is much activity on single organisation based portals which is at odds with our increasingly connected society in the future.

These issues are not a matter of politics. In fact it is vital that they do not become political issues. It is within our gift to put the NHS in everyone's pocket. It is also the greatest birthday present we could give.

The Health Innovation Network has no political affiliations.

6: A SUSTAINABLE SETTLEMENT: LONG-TERM FUNDING FOR THE NHS

Andrew Harrop

Spending on the health service will need to rise by much more than the Conservatives' recently announced plans. But where will the extra funding be found? Tax rises on a scale that the public notice will be required to sustain the NHS. That means a new approach to the way we tax and spend on health.

The National Health Service that Britain loves has grown and flourished for the last 70 years because it has commanded a steadily rising share of the nation's resources. When the NHS was founded in 1948 public spending on healthcare totalled around 3.5 per cent of GDP; by the end of the last Labour government that figure had doubled to around 7 per cent.

As a society we have chosen to spend more on our healthcare because technologies have made more possible; and because we have opted to devote a larger share of our prosperity to good health as we have become richer. Demand for spending has also grown as a result of the nation's changing health and demographic profile. In 1948 people died much earlier; but they tended not to live so long with chronic health conditions which today are a key driver of healthcare spending.

All told, during the first 60 years of the NHS – from 1948 until 2008 – spending increased by an average of 4 per cent a year. This was much more than British economic growth over the period: on average health spending grew 1.3 percentage points faster than GDP each year. But this trend has been broken under Conservative austerity and since 2010 NHS spending has risen by under 1.5 per cent each year on average. It is this that is the root cause of the health service's present challenges and the NHS will thrive only when spending again rises by 4 per cent or more each year. The Conservative party's recent announcement of 5 years' spending growth is not nearly enough.

Over the next decade or two if anything there will be greater pressure to increase spending than over the last 70 years – and not just to undo the damage of the recent squeeze. The annual number of deaths is rising after years of decline; this has spending consequences because the year before death consumes a large proportion of lifetime healthcare costs. In addition, longer periods of disability before death and higher rates of survival into old age mean that many more people are living with long-term health conditions and multiple co-morbidities. It is not even clear that healthier lifestyles will reduce these cost pressures, because they lead to more people living into late old age.

On top of these trends in population health, the pace of innovation in health technologies will certainly be no slower than over the last seven decades and could easily be faster. We can expect to reap the fruits of modern genetic science and constantly accelerating computational power. And unlike in some sectors, new technology in healthcare drives costs up not down, because it makes more possible rather than just reducing the costs of what we already can do. In health, technology does not equate to automation and there are strict limits on the extent to which it is desirable to replace people with machines, when good healthcare depends so much on human relationships.

This is also the reason why over time we cannot expect productivity in healthcare to rise as fast as in the wider economy: in less people-dependent sectors innovation should cut the costs of each unit of activity much more than in health. The last decade has been exceptional in this respect because productivity increases in the NHS have outstripped disastrously weak growth in the private sector. But NHS productivity gains have been unusually high because austerity pressures have led to one-off efficiency savings and this cannot be expected to last.

Productivity improvements will offset some of the upward pressures on NHS spending, but nothing like them all. Current NHS plans which assume annual productivity gains of more than 2 per cent a year are neither plausible nor achievable. They are simply the 'residual' between the amount the service really needs and the amount Conservative ministers have been prepared to give it in recent years. Looking forward, if annual productivity gains are a little under 1 per cent a year – matching the trends of the past 25 years – this should be celebrated as success not written off as failure.

Putting all this together, there are lots of credible independent projections for how much extra spending the NHS will need over the next decade or two. They differ in their methodologies, assumptions and results. But they all tell the same overall long term story, of demand for spending rising by around 4 per cent each year, just like in the health service's first six decades. So the Conservatives' promise of annual rises of 3.4 per cent for the next 5 years is nowhere near enough. One particularly rigorous recent assessment from the Institute for Fiscal Studies and the Health Foundation suggests that NHS revenue spending should rise by 4.7 per cent year for the next five years as 'catch up'. On this basis the Tories' pledge of £20 billion extra by 2023 is a full £9 billion less than what is needed.

And these numbers will be even higher if we do not also invest in social care and other allied services which reduce demand for healthcare. Recent Fabian Society research shows that spending on support and care for older people needs to rise by much more than 4 per cent a year to meet rising demand and plug gaps in today's threadbare services.

The challenge now is to find the money. And after the grinding years of austerity, this is becoming the focus of a new political debate. In the past, NHS increases were often funded by diverting money from other areas of spending – like debt interest, defence and investment. But today there is nowhere left to squeeze and the increases will need to come from higher taxes. Even Conservatives like Theresa May, Jeremy Hunt and Philip Hammond are starting to see that this is inevitable, although it is anathema to their self-image as tax-cutters and state-shrinkers. For the left, tax rises are a more instinctive response, but Labour still needs to proceed cautiously when it comes to raising new revenues on a very large scale.

Whichever side introduces major tax rises, they must either be fairly inconspicuous or command wide public support. 'Inconspicuous' tax increases are those that most people do not notice. They can target fairly small groups (eg raising extra from small numbers of wealthy people, as Labour proposed at the 2017 election). Or they can be invisible to people when the tax change comes (eg freezing the cash value of tax thresholds as the Tories are said to be considering).

Inconspicuous changes along these lines can be used for a few years to raise extra money for health and social care. However sooner or later the scale of spending required means that visible headline tax rates will almost certainly need to rise too, whether that is income tax, national insurance or VAT. Under normal conditions this would stir up public hostility – and for this reason, there is growing political interest in 'hypothecated' or earmarked taxes, to link unpopular tax increase to the NHS which we love and cherish.

This is not a new debate and in 2001 a Fabian Society commission proposed a ringfenced NHS tax. Labour responded with a halfway house solution and in 2002, chancellor Gordon Brown introduced an earmarked rise in national insurance for the NHS, while rejecting a fully hypothecated health tax. With the NHS so close to financial meltdown the case is now even stronger than in the early-2000s for either the Fabian commission's 'hard' hypothecation or Brown's 'soft' version of a one-off earmarked tax rise. The only difference is that these days, most observers would say the funding should cover health and care together.

Permanently ringfenced taxes have the advantage of creating more certainty and transparency. Unlike a single tax hike, they offer a long-term mechanism for generating a steadily rising stream of revenue. By linking health spending to a designated tax base, revenue will expand automatically and at roughly the same pace as rising national prosperity. And when it's known that the money will not be enough over the long-term, planned and clearly explained increases in the earmarked taxes provide a ready-made mechanism to respond to rising needs.

However politicians today should not emulate the last Labour government's choice of the tax to increase. Indeed, looking back with 15 years of hindsight, Labour's decision to use national insurance to pay for health looks very odd, because the tax is paid only by workers and employers. Pensioners who consume around half of all health and social care were therefore exempted from paying more. And turning national insurance into a ring-fenced health tax would not only leave the young paying for the old. It would also finally destroy the contributory principle that links national insurance to the state pension and other earned benefits.

We should be trying to revive not bury this principle to help sustain the state pension's popular support: no one wants to see pensions wither in the same way that other parts of the welfare system have.

A better answer would be to convert a proportion of income tax and VAT into an NHS tax (in England around half of each would cover the costs of the NHS). These health taxes could each be separate and visible on payslips and till receipts, as the point of earmarking is to associate unpopular payments with popular causes (by contrast today virtually nobody knows that up to four pence in every pound of earnings is hypothecated to the NHS via national insurance, because no one is ever told). Other smaller taxes could also be designated as health taxes for example tobacco and alcohol duty and extra taxes might be introduced for social care targeting affluent older people's wealth and non-earnings income.

Such ringfenced health taxes will be resisted by the Treasury as a dangerous innovation. But these ideas are unremarkable in other European countries where healthcare is routinely funded by social insurance or local taxes. And the alternative, of one-off tax rises without an institutional context, is more likely to perpetuate the stop-start spending of recent decades not the sustained long-term growth that health and care so badly needs.

The NHS deserves a long-term investment plan to celebrate its birthday. A one-off spending boost funded by one-off tax rises would offer a temporary solution. But true health taxes might deliver a permanent funding system with both the fiscal buoyancy and public buy-in to meet the nation's demand for rising health-related spending. After years of pain for health and care there should be no taboos on funding. We should debate a new path.

7: PEOPLE FIRST: PUTTING PATIENTS AT THE HEART OF THE HEALTH SERVICE

Chris Graham

The NHS is the institution that makes people most proud to be British. But despite huge advances – and a commitment to listening to patients – workforce pressures too often have a negative impact on staff and patients. To ensure that the NHS remains fit-for-purpose when it reaches its centenary, it must be person-centred in everything it does.

Opening the first NHS hospital in Manchester on 5 July 1948, Nye Bevan described the National Health Service as giving the nation 'the moral leadership of the world'. On other occasions, he described the commitment to providing care free at the point of need for those who required it as 'the most civilised thing in the world'. This is the spirit of the NHS: not merely a system of organising healthcare, but a progressive and revolutionary attempt to create a fairer, better world.

Even more remarkable than the ambitions behind the NHS are the degree to which they have been achieved. Research by the Commonwealth Fund shows that there is less than a 3 per cent difference between high and low earners reporting cost-related access problems to medical care in the UK in 2017 – and even low earners in the UK face fewer financial challenges around health than high earners in the United States. Accordingly, polls routinely show that the NHS is the thing that makes people most proud to be British.

Seventy years on from the creation of the NHS, we live in a more equitable society and enjoy vastly improved health outcomes. But the NHS today faces new challenges, and for our country to retain the moral leadership that Bevan described it must adapt and grow.

Some of the NHS's challenges come, ironically enough, as a direct result of its successes: as a society we are living longer and this means a growing proportion of people are living with multiple long-term conditions and complex care needs. Others reflect broader changes in our society, which is today more diverse and yet more connected than could have been imagined 70 years ago. Together, these changes contribute to vastly increased demand on services, so workloads are growing – and so too are pressures on the doctors, nurses, and other professionals who work on the NHS's frontline.

Funding is, of course, an important part of the challenge. But to ensure that the NHS is fit-for-purpose as a taxpayer-funded health system when it reaches its centenary in 2048, the deeper need is to ensure that the service as a whole is person centred in everything it does.

Long-term conditions

Good healthcare experiences depend on positive therapeutic relationships and interactions between patients and clinicians. Patients tell us that the most important factors for them are clear communication; a sense of being listened to and treated with respect; and the opportunity to be involved in their own care and treatment. Coordination of care is important, especially for those patients with multiple conditions and complex needs.

Traditionally GPs have provided direct relationship continuity by being the first port-of-call for patients, and over the next 30 years they will undoubtedly continue in this role for everyday care needs. But where people need support from a range of different specialists or services – as happens increasingly often – then the challenge is to ensure that sense of continuity and consistency remains.

Our research has shown that people with more complex needs (such as comorbid long-term conditions) report worse experiences of care in the NHS. There are particular challenges where people move between different services, and a common complaint is a feeling of discontinuities in care as people 'slip between the cracks'. Breakdowns in continuity can have repercussions not just for patients and their families but also for other parts of the care system: missed care frequently results in avoidable hospital admissions, increasing demand and service cost.

Addressing this is vital to providing sustainable services that are centred on people's needs. Integrated care systems provide a potential model to tackle this, but their success will depend on a delicate balance of levers and incentives, as well as the local knowledge and expertise to dissolve silos and bring different providers together around a common purpose. The organising principle in all of this must be the patient perspective. Policymakers must ensure that this view is maintained and emphasised at every opportunity.

Putting patients at the centre

Since the NHS Plan in 1996, governments and policymakers have talked about putting patients at the heart of health services. Over the last 20 years, the NHS has led the world in finding new ways to measure and understand people's experiences of care. National surveys of unprecedented scale and reach mean that we have, for more than a decade, been able to track and compare the quality of NHS providers from the patient's perspective, and the information generated has been used extensively to regulate services.

This explosion in measurement has been important in giving leverage to the patient voice and in normalising the idea of patients as active participants in care. The approach is internationally envied and copied, and examples of similar programmes have sprung up across the world.

But measurement has not, to date, led to enough improvement in the quality of services. For example, only 56 per cent of hospital inpatients in 2016 said that they were involved as much as they wanted to be in decisions about their care and treatment – only a modest improvement from 52 per cent 10 years previously in 2006.

With some notable exceptions, many providers have struggled to integrate patient feedback into strategic planning and development. Reasons for this include lack of support from senior leaders; a tendency to view patient experience as a 'nice-to-have' compared to other elements of quality like safety and clinical effectiveness; and a lack of skills and resources to use patient experience information as part of local improvement initiatives. Capacity building work is urgently required to address this. In part this is a question of local funding – but the creation of a national centre of excellence on person centred care should also be considered as a cost-effective means of helping staff across the NHS access the right skills and expertise.

The widespread adoption of digital technologies creates new opportunities to deliver and monitor person centred care. Shared electronic health records should become the norm and will allow patients to lift the veil on clinical records, supporting more open, more equal dialogue between patients and clinicians. The nature of user feedback is changing, too – increasingly discussion between services and their users is becoming open and public through the use of social media platforms like Twitter and Facebook. NHS organisations must respond in kind by showing openness to engaging with patients through these channels.

But digital technologies also create their own challenges around ownership of and access to data – and in the wake of recent scandals the NHS and policymakers must find ways to assure patients about the security and confidentiality of their most sensitive health data. Without public confidence in this, progress towards realising the potential of digital technologies may be cut short.

Looking after staff

Public pride in the NHS is often rooted in positive views of its staff, particularly frontline clinicians. Polling shows that the professionals most widely trusted are nurses and doctors, at 94 per cent and 91 per cent respectively: far ahead of NHS managers at 48 per cent, and more than six times more trusted than politicians. In surveys, the most common types of comments are those praising staff – but all too often this praise is qualified with concerned comments that they 'seemed very stretched' or were 'run off their feet'.

According to the British Social Attitudes survey, the most commonly cited reasons for public dissatisfaction with the NHS are that there are 'not enough staff'; and that 'too little [is] spent' on the service. These views are mirrored in the NHS staff survey, conducted by Picker for NHS England. From more than 480,000 responses, only 31 per cent said that there were enough staff in their organisation for them to do their job properly. And in 2017, the survey showed a six percentage point fall in satisfaction with pay, down from 37 per cent to 31 per cent.

The survey also shows the commitment of healthcare professionals and the sacrifices that they make to maintain a high-quality service. In 2017, 58 per cent of staff said that they regularly worked unpaid additional hours – adding up to an average of around 12 days of unpaid overtime per person per year. This dedication is commendable but not inexhaustible. More than half of all staff (57 per cent) said that within the last three months they had gone to work despite feeling too unwell to perform their duties, and 38 per cent of staff said that they had felt unwell with work related stress in the last 12 months.

Research by Picker and the King's Fund has shown a link between workforce pressures and both staff and patient experience. Hospital trusts with higher sickness absence rates, and where a greater proportion of pay goes to temporary agency staff, have poorer staff and patient experiences. That doesn't mean that agency staff are to blame for poor care or morale – rather that overreliance on temporary staff is no substitute for having a skilled, committed workforce that can buy into an organisation's values and deliver consistent, high-quality care.

The message here is clear: if the NHS is to continue to provide high-quality care for the next 30 years, we need to take care of its staff. This means ensuring that NHS providers have the right number of staff with the right skills – a question both of funding, training, and retaining staff. As Health Education England's recent draft workforce strategy highlighted, the NHS must take a person-centred approach to employment – creating careers rather than jobs, and providing holistic support to help employees thrive and feel valued. After all, happy staff make for happy patients.

A person-centred future

On its 70th birthday, the NHS and its 1.2 million employees can reflect with pride on their achievements. To maintain this pride, and to remain true to the founding spirit of the service, we must strive to ensure that every element of the system is truly person-centred. If this can be achieved, then the NHS can rightly claim to retain the 'moral leadership' that Bevan so eloquently described 70 years ago. But if we falter in this vision, we can expect unmet needs and gaps in provision to grow, threatening the very survival of the service – an outcome that we simply cannot afford.

8: A HUMANE RESPONSE: PUTTING MENTAL WELLBEING AT THE HEART OF THE NHS

Luciana Berger MP

When it comes to attitudes to mental illness, society has come a long way. Yet within the NHS, mental health services are still undervalued and underfunded. A new approach which better addresses the underlying causes of mental ill health would change all of that.

The second half of the twentieth century saw mental health services escape the long, dark shadow cast by Victorian asylums and mental institutions. When the NHS was created 70 years ago, four out of 10 NHS beds were situated in mental health hospitals. Over the next half century, mental health services, apart from in the most acute cases, shifted away from institutions and into the mainstream NHS and the community. This is entirely welcome.

The future must be characterised by a new paradigm shift, tilting our efforts away from treatment and towards prevention of mental illness in the first place. We need a political discourse and a public policy which talks of, and supports, 'mental health' rather than mental illness. Only if we achieve this will we be able to sustain a world-class system of mental health services within the founding ethos of the NHS.

We should be pleased at how far we have come as a society. For centuries, mental ill-health was the cause of fear, misunderstanding, scorn and ridicule. It was a barely understood branch of medicine, with an entirely outmoded language to describe its symptoms and effects. School playgrounds and work canteens rang with phrases such as 'basket cases', 'loony bins', 'psychos' and 'schizos'.

Mental illness was viewed as 'weakness' in men or 'hysteria' in women, and more often than not was the purview of the legal, not the medical, profession. Until just a few years ago, mental illness was a matter of huge stigma, discrimination and prejudice. It could break reputations and trigger loss of status, income and even liberty. People suffering with mental illness were shunned, shunted around the system, or shut away from society.

We should celebrate the campaigners and public figures who have challenged the taboos, often using their own lived experiences, to create a new atmosphere of understanding and acceptance. Just as the language surrounding gender, disability and race has evolved into something more inclusive and less divisive or insulting, so the language associated with mental health has become less stigmatising and raw. A generation of young people are emerging with a better understanding of mental health issues, and a lexicon to describe the concomitant complexities, within a framework of education and health services more attuned to their needs.

This welcome rise of awareness and understanding has not been matched by adequate service improvement. We face a real crisis in our mental health services. Despite the best efforts of thousands of hard-working, dedicated staff, the provision of services is patchy, with long waiting lists and waiting times, and a high threshold to receive services at all. The result is that a patient's condition is left to become more acute before resources are allocated to their treatment: this is both distressing for the individual, and more expensive for the taxpayer. It also has a negative impact on recovery. Services for young people in particular are shamefully inadequate, as the health and social care select committee, on which I serve, has heard from too many witnesses.

Since 2010, we have heard speeches from Conservative prime ministers and government ministers paying lip service to improving mental health. In 2012, after pressure from Labour members of the House of Lords, the coalition government committed to 'parity of esteem' between mental and physical health services. This should have meant that mental health services were equal to the world-class service for physical injury and disease provided by the NHS. But the road to hell is paved with good intentions. The warm words have not been matched by tangible improvements. There are 5,000 fewer mental health nurses now than in 2010. The experiences of patients with a mental illness seeking treatment is so often frustrating. Many incidents of mental illness are simply not diagnosed. Imagine if we treated a patient with cancer or coronary heart disease in the same lackadaisical fashion.

A future Labour government will need to inject more funding into the NHS, just to cope with the rising demands of an ageing population, 'lifestyle' diseases caused by smoking or obesity, and new, expensive technology. A joint report by the Institute for Fiscal Studies and the Health Foundation in May this year found that UK spending on the NHS will have to rise by an average 3.3 per cent a year over the next 15 years to prevent services getting worse, and to improve NHS services for the future, funding increases of 4 per cent a year will be required over the next 15 years. This will require a rebalancing of our system of tax and spend, with those are the top paying more, as part of a fair, progressive system of taxation.

But putting more funding into the NHS is not the answer in itself, especially if funding is soaked up by treating preventable and chronic conditions. If NHS cash is skewed towards physical ailments, the danger is that mental health services remain the Cinderella. The lesson of the last Labour government, which ended in 2010 with the NHS held in the highest public esteem in its history, is that investment must be mirrored by reforms. The real transformation will come when we shift the balance from treatment to prevention.

This prevention agenda must be at the heart of our approach to health and wellbeing, if we want to see the NHS survive on its founding principles, and remain a service used by the vast majority of the population. So how do we prevent mental ill-health? Our understanding of what causes mental illness is developing all the time. It is clear there is a link between certain forms of mental illness and environmental factors, known as the social determinants of health. If we tackle these causes of mental illness, we can prevent many cases from developing in the first place.

For example, we know poor housing, unsafe streets, noisy neighbours, poor air quality, bad diets and financial uncertainty can create the conditions for mental illness to thrive. The uncertainty and dislocation created by the global financial crash has been detrimental to our collective mental health. In coming decades, the upheavals of the technological revolution, the so-called 'fourth industrial revolution', will have a profound effect. These impacts will fall hardest on those in the most precarious settings – people without assets, in low-paid and low-skill jobs, or people without strong social networks and local support. In short, the poorest people will be the hardest hit by change.

As the Mental Health Foundation makes clear, "poverty produces an environment that is extremely harmful to individuals', families' and communities' mental health". There is a clear, causal link between mental ill-health and poverty. Thus, our policies on mental health must be informed by our values of social justice, just as much by medical and psychological considerations.

I have argued, for example in a recent 10-minute rule bill in parliament, that we need to assess every policy against the criteria of whether it enhances or detracts from our nation's physical and mental health. This is sometimes called a 'health in all policies' approach, and it means that no major decision by the next Labour government, or any government, should be made without consideration of how it effects people.

A great Fabian R H Tawney is reputed to have said that there is no greater test of public policy than its impact on the individual. Surely this is correct. The history of public policy is littered with expensive and counter-productive disasters which have added to the public's stress and anxiety. The government's ongoing, shambolic 'reform' of social security is a recent example, with thousands of people thrown into penury and mental ill-health as a result.

A new approach, focused on keeping us mentally and physically well, would avoid these kinds of errors and marshal the whole resource of the state towards a healthy, happy population. It is far too important to be left to a 'director of public health' down a dark town hall corridor, or civil servants ensconced in the labyrinths of Whitehall. It requires all of us to take a collective responsibility for our own wellbeing, matched by a range of public services which are tailored, humane and responsive. This is the 'fully engaged' scenario envisioned by the late Derek Wanless in his landmark report for the last Labour government. He made the stark point that demand will always outstrip supply for healthcare, and the NHS would not be sustainable on then-current projections.

Today, over a decade on from the Wanless report, the issue is even more urgent. We've seen improvements in attitudes, in treatments, and in technology. But we have so much further to go. The clamour of demands on an incoming secretary of state for health will be deafening: more money for A&E, more hospital beds, more doctors and nurses. It is vital that amidst the cacophony there is a still, calm voice arguing for improved mental health services, and for a new focused emphasis on prevention of the causes of mental ill health. This will prove a surer route to save the NHS and create a fairer society than anything else.

9: FIRST CALL: RETHINKING
THE PRIMARY CARE SYSTEM

Paul Williams MP

GPs and other primary care services form the frontline of the NHS. But they are now under huge pressure and often unable to make the investments which could benefit the health of the communities they serve. A new approach to primary care could offer the opportunity for change, putting the focus firmly on prevention rather than cure.

Primary care has been an integral part of the first 70 years of the NHS. Although GPs, community pharmacists, dentists and opticians don't usually work directly for NHS organisations, they carry, as contractors, the trusted NHS 'brand'. They provide universal services to millions of people every day.

Primary care frames care for an individual in a uniquely important way. It does so through a lens which sees much more than a disease – it views a person in the context of their family, their work, their home and their community.

General practices are at the heart of primary care. GPs hold a contract with the NHS to provide services to patients on their list. They should be available to their patients who are, or who believe themselves to be, ill. More than 99 per cent of the population are registered with a GP.

There are many strengths to our system of primary care. As the NHS changes to adapt to the future, it is crucial to retain these assets. Probably the strongest element is the workforce – thousands of doctors, nurses, managers and receptionists who serve patients beyond their contracted duties and hours. The commitment of staff, the flexibility to change quickly and the fact that primary care teams know, understand and provide on-going care for their patients make UK general practice second to none.

However, there are also weaknesses to the current model, including the dilemma of continuity of care versus accessibility for patients; problems with workforce recruitment, retention and development and the difficulty of encouraging all general practices to take on some NHS work, adopt technologies and make investments when their own organisations may not realise the benefits. Addressing these weaknesses will be crucial in ensuring the NHS is fully equipped for the next 70 years.

Continuity of care versus accessibility

A universal service should be there for everyone, but not the same for everyone. If you are frail, or have long-term conditions, then it is likely that your care will be best delivered by someone who knows you well. You will get care without having to explain your problems to people who don't know you, will design your care with someone experienced in the health problems you have, and they will make better decisions about the involvement of other services in your care. It may be better to wait a few days for an appointment with this team – as it is not possible for the people who know you best to be at work seven days a week.

But for other people, the priority is to get care as quickly and conveniently as possible. It does not matter so much to them who provides that care.

Our current model of general practice has prioritised continuity of care for all. But with part-time working and the advent of a seven-day-a-week service this isn't now possible.

Although continuity is vital for some people, for working families and younger people sometimes accessibility trumps continuity.

Some groups of general practices are starting to use data to 'segment' their patient populations. Patients with the most complex needs are prioritised for continuity. They need a relationship with a health professional they know more than anything else. And those who want to be seen as quickly and conveniently as possible and are likely to need care as a single episode get a different service that prioritises accessibility.

Workforce recruitment, retention and development

General practice is a doctor-dominated service. In most practices, unlike in hospitals, there are more doctors than other clinical staff. But general practice is struggling to recruit and sickness, retirement and poor morale are all putting pressure on the current model. Sometimes when a one member of staff is absent in a small practice a group of patients don't get their care until he or she returns. Departures can leave doctors fearful of being the 'last man standing'.

Future general practice will need to be larger. It is said that the ideal size of organisation is large enough to withstand a couple of departures and a few people on long-term sick leave, but small enough so that everyone knows each other at the Christmas party. This probably means an optimum size of 30,000 to 50,000 patients per primary care organisation.

There are also many more opportunities in primary care to expand the workforce beyond the medical model. Pharmacists, physiotherapists and nurses have all been welcomed into many practices. Some have taken this a step further and have GPs working like hospital consultants, overseeing a team of professionals. Strong nurse leadership can bring more nurses into primary care, ensure less variation in quality between practices and a create more opportunities for learning and career progression. Social prescribing creates a box of new tools to help improve health.

Encouraging all general practices to invest

Before I entered parliament, as well as practicing as a GP, I worked as a commissioner of services and later as the leader of a GP federation. Even when it was clearly in the interests of patients to deliver care from their local general practice, it wasn't easy or sometimes even possible to change the system to get this outcome.

Under existing contractual relationships, much of the 'extra' work that might be suited to be delivered in the community is optional for GPs. There is a real tension between some practices who want to take on extra work and expand their 'business' and others who feel overwhelmed by the existing work that they do and have no desire to commit to anything extra. GPs have to choose between the interests of their patients and the interests of their business.

This results in a strategic paralysis. If commissioners are not able to persuade all general practices in their local area to deliver new community-based care then they cannot get a service for their whole population. It also means the 'price' of commissioning from primary care isn't always good value for money.

GPs should be embracing change, but the current model of general practice does not always adopt new technologies. Uptake of electronic consultations has been frustratingly slow. Technology that might enable patients to have blood tests analysed in the practice, or get instant cardiac investigations does not get used because it would cost a practice to invest in them – with an impact on the 'profit' that GP partners take – and any savings would be realised by a different part of the NHS.

Small practices have little incentive to take on the costs of training and developing staff, as there is a risk that they will train an individual who will take their new skills to a different organisation.

What does a great solution look like?

Prevention really is better than cure. We have the knowledge to be able to keep people well, healthy and usually out of hospital. To rise to the challenge of demography and to provide the greatest opportunity to keep people well, the NHS has to make the strategic shift away from reactive acute hospital services and towards proactive community-based care.

Most NHS trusts are hospital trusts or mental health trusts – organisations that are usually very good at what they do, but not specialists in prevention, early detection and keeping people well in their communities. The experts in non-hospital care are GPs. But they still work in small organisations without the capacity or the incentive to run population-level prevention and community-based healthcare programmes. Community services are often run by acute hospitals as an add-on to their core work.

There are few NHS community providers in England, and none that currently include all GPs working together with community nurses, mental health services and social care. One solution to some of these problems is to form a GP federation – bringing GPs practices together – but these are still non-NHS organisations and all but the bravest GPs are resisting pooling their contracts

There is a strong case for larger primary care organisations working within the NHS. They need to be big enough to be able to provide a universal service that offers different types of care to different patients and strong enough to challenge the power of large hospital trusts and stop the flow of resources away from prevention and into reaction. They also need to be attractive enough for the very best clinical and managerial staff to build careers in and independent enough to remove any profit motive from GPs and encourage investment in technology and community-based services. But at the moment these organisations do not exist.

The NHS of the future needs these more powerful organisations with real expertise and resources to run out-of-hospital care. On the 70th birthday of the NHS, it is time to complete the work done in 1948 and bring general practice firmly into the NHS, within out-of-hospital care organisations incorporating general practice, community nursing and mental healthcare.

If social care were added in then new integrated care trusts (ICTs), working in partnership with the voluntary and community Sector could deliver free-at-the-point-of-need integrated health and social care services to entire populations.

Integrated care trusts could eventually hold the whole local NHS budget, investing in prevention and incurring 'cost' when an individual needed an acute hospital admission. Realigning the incentives to encourage a social model of healthcare would utilise the resources of a whole community to keep people well, reducing demand on medical services. This, in turn, creates more time for medical services to provide high quality care. Patients would see powerful, effective primary care and the health and care service would realise the previously elusive strategic shift from cure to prevention.

10: STAFFING MATTERS: ENSURING A MODERN AND SKILLED WORKFORCE

Sara Gorton

Healthcare staff are the heart of the NHS. We need to ensure that we value the role they play and create the conditions to allow them to can offer the highest quality of care. Tackling staff shortages, cracking down on bullying and offering good routes for progression will all need to be part of the package.

The 70th anniversary of the creation of the NHS is without a doubt a huge cause for celebration – for patients and staff alike. The health service continues to be the envy of the world – revered both for its equity of access and its efficient delivery of services.

The healthcare workforce is rightly lauded for its role in this success story. The majority of the NHS budget goes on staffing costs, but the public considers this money well spent. Opinion polls continue say that nurses and doctors are the professions they trust the most.

But staffing issues have recently become the top concern for those charged with managing care in hospitals. This should come as no surprise. The past few years have seen a great deal of upheaval within the NHS and frequent attempts at major service redesign – some more successful than others. Yet this has all taken place without any coherent overall workforce strategy. Strategic workforce planning seems to have become anathema in the NHS, certainly since Andrew Lansley's disastrous Health and Social Care Act of 2012.

So it was a welcome first move when late last year Health Education England produced a draft health and care workforce strategy. It is hoped that at the time of writing, this is being strengthened considerably into a more robust statement of what is required to develop and sustain a modern healthcare workforce for the next decade and beyond.

At its most basic, a modern healthcare workforce is one where there is enough staff to guarantee patient safety and where employees are confident they can deliver the highest quality of service for those they care for.

And yet this is clearly not the case at the moment. The number one reason given by the public for dissatisfaction with the health service is that there aren't enough staff. The figures bear this out. More than 8 per cent of NHS posts are vacant, including one in 10 nursing roles. Respondents to UNISON surveys repeatedly point to there being insufficient levels of staffing to guarantee safe, dignified and compassionate care on wards.

There are many reasons for these shortages. Nearly a decade of cuts has wiped thousands of pounds off the value of health workers' pay packets and has led to excessive workloads becoming the norm for most. This has badly damaged morale within the sector, with thousands of staff voting with their feet by leaving permanent employment to take on agency work or quitting the NHS completely.

These problems have been exacerbated by the government's inability to provide sufficient reassurances to EU nationals in the workforce ahead of the UK's exit from Europe. Taken together, these failures threaten to choke off the traditional supply of international workers who have, almost from day one, helped rescue the NHS from its perennial staffing shortages.

There is still no sign that the government understands the severity of the situation. The abolition of the bursary for healthcare students threatens to cut further still the supply of nurses, midwives and other health professionals to the NHS for years to come.

One way of offering reassurances to patients and staff would be to legislate for safe staffing levels, as has already taken place in Wales. For this to have the greatest possible impact, the system should also develop tools for assessing the level of work that each member of staff can reasonably be expected to undertake. That's because safe staffing levels are only meaningful if there are also robust processes for measuring workload levels.

Of course extra staff have to be paid for. It is not possible to have a modern healthcare workforce without substantial and sustained investment.

The government has indicated it will produce a longer term funding settlement for the NHS. But this will only prove successful if the increases are sufficient to bring the health service back up to the sort of funding levels it enjoyed for the first 60 years of its existence. Ideally this would be funding comparable to France and Germany, which each spend a considerably larger proportion of their GDP on healthcare.

There are other problems too that the NHS needs to overcome before it can be considered a model employer. Frequent surveys, including recent work from UNISON, have shown that violence and harassment continues to be a real problem, experienced by far too many staff. The NHS must strive to be an employer that enforces a rigorous zero-tolerance approach to the abuse of its staff.

The NHS also needs to do more to tackle bullying and harassment. The NHS has lasted for 70 years because at its heart are the basic values of fairness and equality. But these must apply equally to its staff. Unfortunately the latest annual NHS staff survey shows there's been a rise in discrimination at work. It is completely unacceptable that black and minority ethnic staff continue to be treated unfavourably in the workplace and that disabled nurses are faced with concerns about a lack of progression opportunities and find job offers being withdrawn.

NHS England has begun work to tackle discrimination through the workforce race equality standard and the workforce disability equality standard, but UNISON is now calling for a unified equality standard to bring together these and other strands of work. The NHS needs a coherent whole-system plan for boosting equality and diversity in the NHS that will benefit both staff and the patients they care for.

Looking to the future, more can and should be done to ensure that plans for new routes into healthcare roles live up to their potential. The delay in getting nursing apprenticeships off the ground has been a particular cause for concern. These could provide a lifeline for aspiring nurses who find themselves priced out of the traditional student route by the replacement of bursaries with tuition fees.

The NHS also needs urgent action to restore continuing professional development funding, with national budgets having been cut by more than 60 per cent since 2015. This is another factor that contributes to the demoralisation of the workforce and ultimately has the potential to affect the quality of care that patients receive.

A lack of training is something that particularly affects those staff at lower pay bands. Agenda for Change is the national pay scale for all NHS staff, excluding doctors, dentists and most senior managers. It is estimated that staff in bands 1–4 are responsible for more than half of direct patient contact, yet they benefit from only around 5 per cent of the whole training budget.

This speaks to a wider concern that too often support service staff are undervalued and underrecognised within the NHS. The health service is about more than just doctors and nurses, essential though they are. The non-clinical work-force – such as cleaners, porters, catering staff, managers, administrative staff and IT workers – is central to the smooth running of the NHS. Yet these workers are all too often seen as an easy target for cuts or outsourcing.

The most recent example of this is the current trend for trusts to set up wholly owned subsidiary companies and transfer services like estates and facilities management to them. Apart from directly affecting the terms and condi-tions of new staff that start working for these organisations, this approach creates barriers between different parts of the healthcare team. It also fails to recognise the great pride staff feel in wearing the NHS logo on their uniforms and working for the nation's most popular organisation.

Finally, there is a need for a greater recognition of the positive role that unions can play in our NHS. In part this is through ensuring that the workforce voice informs partner-ship working with employers and government. The fact that the NHS Social Partnership Forum has endured – despite the upheavals and reorganisation of the past eight years – is testament to the benefits this way of working brings for employers, staff and the wider NHS.

But the importance of unions is not restricted to partner-ship working. Unions also play an important role in the development of staff, with many providing their own train-ing for members. At a time when training budgets have been cut, this can be invaluable for employers in boosting the skills and morale of their workforce.

So, as the NHS reaches 70, healthcare staff will be the first to celebrate the longevity of the UK's most cherished national institution. But to guarantee another 70 years, the NHS must ensure that addressing the many pressing work-force concerns is right at the top of its to-do list.

11: LEARNING LESSONS: PUTTING THE NHS BACK IN PUBLIC HANDS

John Lister

The history of private sector involvement in the NHS has been a troubled one. There is evidence that the mood is changing. But more needs to be done to bring services back in-house and to ensure that the fragmentation which has so damaged the NHS comes to an end.

Britain's NHS is celebrating its 70th anniversary this year, but for fully half of that time our health service has been battered and distorted by ill-conceived efforts to open up contracts for private providers.

The 35 year-long catalogue of private sector failures is unbroken and still growing – yet even now a minority of neoliberal privatisers keeps plugging away in the hopes that somehow eventually one of their plans will work out. It is time to draw a line under this sorry episode.

Unlike some of the utilities that were publicly flogged off in the 1980s by Margaret Thatcher, the NHS is loved as an institution. Its creation meant that healthcare in Britain – unlike nationalised electricity, gas or telephones – ceased to be a commodity or service to be paid for by those who could afford it. For the first time anywhere, healthcare became free to all at point of use, funded from general taxation, and delivered on the basis of clinical need, not ability to pay. GP services, hospital care, prescriptions, dental care and opticians were all covered.

Other than a handful of back woods Conservative reactionaries, no MP since then has hankered to bring back the system of charges to see a GP, charges for hospital treatment, or the limited workplace insurance system that existed before the NHS.

The private healthcare sector itself has shown no interest in taking over the sectors of the NHS which offer high risk but little or no profit – and that refers to most of the service: there have been no suggestions since 1948 of any company wanting to take over NHS in-patient medical cases, emergency services, complex surgery, most mental health services or maternity. So it is safe to say that there will never be any NHS equivalent to the 1980s 'tell Sid' campaign adverts which promoted the sale of shares in the gas industry. Privatisation of healthcare has had to be done on the sly, out of the public eye, piecemeal, by manoeuvre and through apparently obscure 'reform'.

Efforts at privatising the provision of non-clinical services began under Thatcher in 1983–4 with competitive tendering of contracts for hospital cleaning and other ancillary services – with ministers pressing for contracts to go to the cheapest bid. This opened up crucial services to cheapskate companies that were eager to cut staff numbers, hours, pay and conditions, in order to scrape a profit from already low-paid staff and underfunded services.

As unions and campaigners had warned, this type of 'competition' – a race to the bottom – had predictable results: it drove down the quality of services, and drove away many of the dedicated NHS staff who had previously been part of ward teams, but now found themselves ruthlessly exploited and unable to do the job properly for patients. Hygiene standards collapsed, MRSA and other hospital-acquired infections began to spread – along with contract failures and scandals.

Thatcher went on to create an 'internal market' within the NHS, separating out 'purchasers' (health authorities and large GP practices) from 'providers' – the hospitals and other services, which were obliged to 'opt out' of health authority control to become NHS trusts and compete for contracts to treat patients. This created a new and costly layer of bureaucracy and an alien language of 'entrepreneurialism.' Thatcher pulled short of any attempt to privatise the provision of clinical care.

In 1992, Tory chancellor Norman Lamont set out proposals for new hospitals and other public sector investment to be funded through the private finance initiative (PFI), a system summarised by his successor Kenneth Clarke as 'privatising the provision of capital'.

However, no hospital PFI deals were signed until Labour – which initially opposed the idea – embraced it as a plank of Tony Blair's New Labour manifesto. From 1997 a rapid succession of PFI deals were signed – paying vastly inflated bills over 30 years or more for the building of hospitals that were often too small, on hard to access sites, poorly designed, and short of beds. PFI has become a by-word for poor value and rip-offs by tax-dodging offshore companies.

From 2000, alongside increased spending on the NHS, health secretary Alan Milburn and his successors began experimenting with privatisation of clinical care. A concordat was signed with private hospitals to take on excess elective operations from NHS trusts, which were to be paid for by the NHS at eye-wateringly high costs. Independent sector treatment centres were commissioned: in which overseas companies, delivered uncomplicated elective surgery – costing an average 11 per cent more than NHS trusts.

Any government addressing the problems of privatisation needs to come to grips with the scale of the problems with their roots in the 2000s. Private companies were brought in to deliver MRI scans and even GP services: The Department of Health set up a commercial directorate. NHS chief executive Nigel Crisp in 2005 unveiled plans for 'world class commissioning,' even offering community health service contracts to 'any willing provider'.

Needless to say, none of these schemes, which consistently undermined the viability of NHS trusts, have proved value for money. The Commons Health Committee concluded in 2010 that: "After 20 years of costly failure, the purchaser/provider split may need to be abolished."

Nonetheless when the Conservative-led coalition took office in 2010 after the banking crash, they showed within weeks they had learned nothing from previous failures. A hitherto concealed white paper proposed a massive top-down reorganisation of the NHS – to more firmly entrench a competitive market, hand more of the NHS budget to private providers – and expand private wings of foundation trusts.

The resulting Health and Social Care Act (2012) has served only to further fragment and disorganise the NHS, putting inexperienced GPs onto the boards of 211 clinical commissioning groups, which are required by the Act to put an ever larger range of services out to tender. Many have done so – and many have failed.

The largest failures have been five-year contracts for older people's services in Cambridgeshire and cancer services in Staffordshire. In each case, most private bidders withdrew – convinced they could make no profit. The cancer contract was awarded to a consortium led by private contractor Interserve, only to be withdrawn again as it became clear they could not deliver. The Cambridgeshire contract collapsed within eight months.

There have also been failures all over the country in patient transport services, where a number of companies won contracts they could not deliver. A lucrative seven-year

£700m contract for GP practice support went to high-profile contractor Capita, whose reorganisation effectively wrecked the previous system and axed jobs, but has since delivered only failure.

Recent figures from NHS Providers show private firms have won a larger share than NHS trusts of the smallest contracts in community health services (amounting to just 5 per cent of total annual contract value), but delivered none of the promised improvements in quality. By contrast all of the bigger, riskier community health contracts have attracted only NHS bids.

It is worrying that despite the mounting evidence that private provision of services represents poor value, the figures show levels of spending on private clinical providers have doubled since 2010. However private spending is still a small component (less than 8 per cent) of NHS spending, and the rate of growth has slowed. Some of this spending is from NHS providers paying to use private hospitals, mental health facilities and diagnostic services to bridge gaps in NHS capacity created by the eight-year cash squeeze which has forced the closure of thousands of acute and mental health beds since 2010.

There is evidence that the mood is changing. In the past three years, the rhetoric from NHS England, and from many NHS managers has markedly changed.

No official policy documents now argue the merits of competition for NHS contracts. Even the academics have given up the hopeless quest for evidence that it delivers the claimed cost reductions, quality improvements and efficiency. Bitter experience over 35 years has proved the opposite is the case.

New Labour's insistence that 'patient choice' had to be central has been eclipsed by austerity cuts throwing doubt on the system's ability to satisfy the most universal 'choice' – for easy access to good, safe hospital services. Instead there is a new management focus on talk of 'integration', 'collaboration' and 'systems' – all of which fly in the face of the purchaser/provider split and competition. If trusts and CCGs seriously want 'integration' they must halt the process of disintegration.

Opposition to privatisation is therefore not ideological, but practical. The private sector delivers cost savings only at the expense of quality, and offers no useful expertise.

The 2012 Act, which even Conservatives now see as a disaster, must be repealed. The public, who never supported the Act, will readily support moves to put the NHS back together again, as long as it is properly funded, values staff, and begins to work coherently as a system.

Many are rightly suspicious of NHS claims to favour 'accountable care' and 'integrated care' organisations while the Act is still in force and private profiteers like Virgin are still pressing for contracts. Scrapping the Act would open up a proper discussion about how best to plan and organise services after 30 years of division, focused on patients, not profits: on healthcare, not ideology. It will take time to put things right.

Buy-outs of privatised contracts can be expensive: but services can be brought back in-house as contracts expire. If companies are persuaded there will be no profits to make up for their loss-leader contracts they may cut their losses and walk away.

Staff in privatised services must be assured that the NHS will both bring services back in-house and also invest in staff and resources to restore high standards. Meanwhile they must be encouraged to work with campaigners to expose private sector failures.

Trusts must also be forced to stop their ill-conceived moves to hive off support staff into 'wholly owned companies' outside the NHS. The best managers already know that the only way to restore the health of our NHS is to regain control over services that have been damaged by fragmentation, and empower staff once more to collaborate and work as NHS teams.

We have had to learn these lessons the hard way, from the serious errors of the last 35 years. It would not only be madness, but hypocritical and evasive for a future government to make the same mistakes again. We now need people to see Labour committed to ensure we never stray back down the dead end of privatisation, and to restore the NHS as a public service, publicly owned, free, for all, for ever.

ENDNOTES

'An equal stake?'

1   Daly G., Jesson J. and Gulliver K. (forthcoming) The Power of Place: Health Inequalities, Housing and Community in the West Midlands Conurbation with a Foreword by Professor Sir Michael Marmot, Director of the Institute of Health Equity.

Structural issues

2   Whilst there are clearly benefits in the current plans to align NHSE and NHSI (https://improvement.nhs.uk/documents/2823/Next_steps_on_aligning_the_work_of_NHS_England_and....pdf), I cannot see the organisational logic in merging them. The current problems of overlap reflects the lack of clarity in their roles.

3   The currently envisaged regional structure is based around seven regions. There are many different permutations being discussed. What matters is that there is alignment.

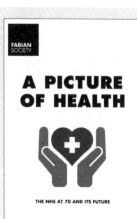

A picture
of health
The NHS at 70
and its future

How to use this discussion guide

The guide can be used in various ways by Fabian local
societies, local political party meetings and trade union
branches, student societies, NGOs and other groups.

- You might hold a discussion among local members
  or invite a guest speaker – for example, an MP, aca-
  demic or local practitioner to lead a group discussion.

- Some different key themes are suggested. You might
  choose to spend 15–20 minutes on each area, or
  decide to focus the whole discussion on one of the
  issues for a more detailed discussion.

A discussion could address some or all of the
following questions:

1. Within a few years of its creation, the NHS had become,
   as Bevan so eloquently put it, part of the texture of
   our national life. It still stands as the expression of
   our national values. In a changing world, how can
   we ensure that it remains so for the next 70 years?

2. The NHS reforms enacted by the coalition government
   caused huge upheaval and discontent and many have
   argued we should resist further wholesale change.
   But given the challenges the health service faces,
   is it now time to revisit the reform agenda?

3. The NHS will need a significant increase in funding
   over the next few years. Is a hypothecated health tax
   the answer? Would it make taxpayers value the health
   service more – or make it easier for its critics to argue
   that a publicly funded NHS is too expensive?

4. Is there ever a case for private sector involvement
   in the NHS?

Please let us know what you think

Whatever view you take of the issues, we would very
much like to hear about your discussion. Please send
us a summary of your debate (perhaps 300 words)
to info@fabians.org.uk
